THE PROBLEM—
AND THE ANSWER

GW00838588

My Hay I

I expect you have been through the wretched business of going on a diet, losing half a stone (maybe even more) and then, unable to sustain the starvation program, *bingeing* and putting all the weight back on again plus a bit more.

You can put an end to all that, AND lose weight if you are overweight, AND be more healthy, AND enjoy your food!

My simplified version of the Hay diet food combining system is not a 3-day wonder but a way of life. It starts to work remarkably quickly, and the benefits to your figure, looks, health and energy should be rapid, surprising, and permanent. You eat *plenty* — including butter, cream and wine!

By this I mean that you are not endlessly *trying to cut down* — 'I mustn't eat this or that' — but instead you'll have feelings like 'Gosh, I'm hungry! When's lunch?'. You then eat *plenty at that meal*.

CHRISTINE RICHMOND
Llanfihangel, 1994

CONTENTS

What if I Fail?

If you are eating out, if you are tempted, or if you are just a bit depressed and you 'simply can't resist' a bit of a blow-out, have you failed?

No, you haven't! You go straight back to the Hay diet at the very next meal and carry on as normal.

What you do *not* do is starve for a day in penitence, or live off half a grapefruit and a lettuce leaf a day for a week!

Lapses will become less and less frequent the longer you are on the Hay diet. They will occur — we are but human. But be assured, a prompt return to the Hay diet will hold you right.

SUCCESS will fuel your determination. You will find it more and more easy to choose the right things from whatever goodies are on offer, and less and less easy to give way to temptations.

This way you NEVER fail.

The Diet Explained

THE BASIC DIET CONSISTS OF —

ONE *STARCH*

ONE *PROTEIN*

and ONE *ALKALI-FORMING*

MEAL A DAY

THE AIM IS TO SEPARATE FOODS WHICH REQUIRE DIFFERENT ENZYMES FOR THEIR DIGESTION.

THIS MEANS KEEPING *PROTEINS* SEPARATED FROM *STARCHES*.

SOME FOODS ARE *NEUTRAL* AND MAY BE EATEN WITH EITHER PROTEINS OR STARCHES.

NB Notice in which columns of the Chart, pages 6-7, the various **fruits** are listed.

IT'S AS SIMPLE AS THAT!

HOW TO START
for Slimmers

STAGE 1

1

Without making **any other changes** to the food you eat, simply separate **proteins** from **starches.** The Chart on pages 6 and 7 explains these.

Your meals will now be *'Protein-based'* or *'Starch-based'*. (*'Neutrals'* may be eaten with any meal.)

You will start to lose weight as a result of simply making this one change — men especially. It should not take above a week to learn to sort out the two main food types.

Make sure you leave **The Gap** (page 13) — at least 4 hours between meals of different food types. This is **vital** if the diet is to work.

STAGE 2

2

Study the list of **alkali**-forming foods on page 4.

Increase the amount of these foods in **all** your meals, while keeping the *Protein-based* and the *Starch-based* meals separate **and** making sure of the 4-hour **gap** between them.

How to Start for Slimmers continues on page 5

The Alkali-forming foods

Some foods are Alkali-forming, some are acid-forming.

One pure-alkali-forming meal should be eaten

each day

— but still keep the *proteins* separate from the *starches*.

The Alkali-forming foods are —

- **FRUITS**, including bananas.
- **DRIED FRUITS**.
- **NUTS**, almonds, brazils and hazelnuts.
- **SALADS** and **HERBS.**
- **VEGETABLES**, green and root.
- **POTATOES**, especially in their jackets.
- **MILLET.**

Alkali-forming foods **should provide about 80% of our diet**. Some alkali-forming foods are STARCH, some PROTEIN, and some are NEUTRAL, so they are normally scattered among your starch and protein meals. Consider this when you look at what is on your plate.

NB Yoghurt, wheatgerm, butter, and oil may be added to alkali-forming meals.

HOW TO START
for Slimmers

STAGE 3

Introduce one **purely** *Alkali-forming* meal each day, based on either fruit or potatoes or salads. A fruit breakfast is probably the easiest way to do this, *eg:*

> Fresh orange juice,
> Sliced fruits,
> with one tablespoon of wheatgerm, plus yoghurt.

STAGE 4

Settle down to the daily meals routine of

> One **purely** *Alkali-forming* ,
> One *Starch-based*, and
> One *Protein-based.*

Have them in any order that suits you. Change the order as often as you like.

STAGE 5

Now you are fully on the Hay diet. Check carefully through the list on page 8 and improve the quality of every meal.

And remember, page 4 is vital to success.

THE HAY DIET CHART

Protein ——— Neutral ——— Starch

Protein

All meats

Fish

Shellfish

Poultry

Game

Eggs

Cheese

Milk

Yoghurt

* All fresh FRUIT

Neutral

Notes

1 Neutral foods may be eaten with protein *OR* starch.

2 The *Alkali-forming* foods are marked * .

* All VEGETABLES *except*
the 'potato group' (see under Starch)

* All SALADS, including avocado, sprouted legumes & seeds

* Herbs and spices

Butter & cream

Cream cheese

Starch

* Potatoes

* Sweet potatoes

* Jerusalem artichoke

* Pumpkin

* *ALL alkali-forming*
Bananas, dates, figs, currants, sultanas raisins (and grapes, pears and paw-paw — only if *very* sweet)

Cereals
Grain, rice etc

		Bread
Dried apricots	Sunflower, safflower, and sesame oils	Flour
		Oatmeal
Dried beans, dried peas, lentils etc. *(use sparingly as these are high in both protein and starch)*	Egg yolk	Milk & yoghurt (use sparingly)
	* Nuts (<u>not</u> peanuts)	
	* Seeds & raisins	
	Wheatgerm, bran, oatgerm	
Dry wines & dry cider	Whisky & gin	**Beer and Ale**

Sugar substitutes	Maple syrup, a little honey or honey water, concentrated apple juice, orange juice, raisins.
Salad dressings	Oil, lemon, mustard, salt & pepper. Oil & garlic, salt & pepper. Oil, cider vinegar, garlic, mustard, salt & pepper. Home-made mayonnaise & cream dressings. Soy sauce.

Special Pointers
for Slimmers

1 **FATS Butter, cream and cheeses**.
   Limit these to TWO OUNCES (50 gm) per day. Use low fat, live yoghurt — it helps.

2 **SUGARS** including **hidden sugars** in manufactured foods. *CUT DOWN RELENTLESSLY; they are making you fat!*

3 **STARCHES** *Eat jacket potatoes and wholegrain rice in preference to bread and cereals. AVOID refined flours and cereals.*

4 **PROTEINS** *Limit red meat to twice a week, and don't take large helpings of any main protein food. Eat plenty of veg. and fruit.*

5 **RAW FOOD** *Eat PLENTY of fruit, salads and RAW vegetables.*

6 **NUTS & DRIED FRUIT** *Excellent, but don't overindulge (Avoid peanuts).*

7 **ALCOHOL** *Beer, ale and lager are LOADED with sugar and strictly OFF LIMITS for slimmers. Stick to dry wines, and the occasional Scotch or Gin.*

8 **SALT** *Be very careful. We all ADD too much.*

9 **HUNGER** *WAIT TILL YOU ARE REALLY HUNGRY!*

10 **ALWAYS check with your Doctor** before making any change to your diet.

Addiction

I can almost hear you thinking, "What about my daily craving for chocolate?" — or breakfast cereals, biscuits, cream cakes, sugary beverages, or whatever.

Just follow the diet! Don't worry about them!
AS THE ALKALI-FORMING FOODS ARE INCREASED, THE CRAVINGS WILL VANISH!

Meanwhile, when you are tempted, make sure that these indulgences are eaten ONLY in connection with a STARCH meal.

Trust in the diet and the addictions will quietly drop away. Put the effort into making sure you are getting the diet right, NOT into *trying* to stop your cravings.

Correct Food In Store

Don't let yourself down by not having plenty of Hay diet foods in the house.

See   *'My Hay Diet Pocketbook'*
        — page 8, **Shopping**.

Exercise

DON'T !!

I can think of nothing more stupid than an overweight person out jogging or puffing their way through a forced exercise program.

Extra exercise makes you *very* hungry for *all* foods.

As you lose weight on the Hay diet your new-found energy will make you more active anyway. Once you are losing weight, then is the time to start an exercise or body-building program, NOT BEFORE!

So Exercise Programs along with Crash Diets are **OUT**. Candlelit dinners and relaxation are **IN**.

Shape

You will notice after a few weeks on the Hay diet that your shape has changed, and for the better!

This may not coincide with any particular weight loss, but it always happens. Others will notice and probably comment!

Hunger

If you become *very hungry*, have an extra **starch meal**. Starches for such an emergency include —

popcorn,

a potato dish,

cooked rice with raisins and peppers,

mashed banana with yoghurt and maple syrup.

The emergency must not become a habit!

Make sure you eat plenty at main meals

Make one meal a day a feast of 3 courses, *eg* —

A *starter* of grapefruit, avocado, shellfish, or soup;

Main dish, a protein, with a sauce and 3 veg.

A *pud,* fruit salad or strawberries with cream and/or yoghurt.

Plus wine and 'proper' coffee.

Hunger Suppressants in whatever form are very, very dangerous.

The chemicals and processing used in the manufacture of most Soft Margarines, Instant Coffee, Decaffeinated Coffee, and Artificial Sweeteners are **better avoided**.

The Wheatgerm Trick

This is a marvellous help. Have a small quantity of wheatgerm every day — with every meal (at home) if you like. It can be treated as a little 'extra' to the normal diet meals.

Put 2 teaspoons of wheatgerm into a small bowl, add yoghurt and a little maple syrup.

Wheatgerm seems to calm the whole digestive system, which in turn calms you and helps you to maintain the diet.

Buy wheatgerm in small quantities and keep it in the fridge. Most supermarkets and health-food stores stock it.

The Gap

This is probably *the* most important point for slimmers —

Eat *plenty* at your main meals *and* —

Be *very strict* with yourself about leaving a FULL 4-HOUR **GAP** BETWEEN MEALS.

You can then look forward to your next large meal.

Tea-time is the danger-zone! If the Gap between lunch and your evening meal is over-long, 4 hours after lunch (not less), either have —

a) *If the evening meal is to be PROTEIN,*
Fresh fruit salad and yoghurt, or —

b) *If the evening meal is to be STARCH,*
Raw muesli soaked in water (preferably the bottled, still kind) with raisins, seeds, yoghurt and a little maple syrup or molasses, or a small roll with cream cheese and salad.

Commuters may not be able to do any of these, though salad rolls should be easy enough (but only before a starch meal). Think ahead to what your evening meal will be and choose appropriately from the Chart, pages 6-7. Even a bag of nuts (NOT peanuts!) and raisins and a scotch would be fine — all are Neutral.

Results

For anyone *really, honestly* following my simplified Hay diet food combining system

    — keeping the *proteins* separate from the *starches*

    — checking the *gap* between meals

    — and eating plenty of *alkali-forming* foods

the results are ***STUNNING !***

The Hay diet method is totally self-correcting — weight for height. You needn't even weigh yourself — just look in the mirror. The mirror will show you that the results are a success. Give your bathroom scales away, or hide them in the furthest corner of the attic.

Remember, today's energy comes from yesterday's food. What you are eating *now* will determine your energy level, looks *and weight* for tomorrow. So —

    SLIM ! — Don't *Starve and binge!*
    Start on my simplified Hay diet...
    Eat PLENTY of food
    ENJOY IT
    IMPROVE YOUR LOOKS
    ENJOY LIFE!